RISE UP

AND

$\mathscr{B}$UILD

GOOD HEALTH

Practical Insights To Heal Your Emotions by Healing Your Body

DANA RONGIONE

RISE UP
AND
$\mathscr{B}$UILD
GOOD HEALTH

*Practical Insights To Heal
Your Emotions by Healing Your Body*

DANA RONGIONE

All Scripture notations are taken from
The Holy Bible, KJV.

Disclaimer: The purpose of this book is to educate. The review of personal experience is presented for informational purposes only. This book should not be used as a basis for self-diagnosis or treatment without first consulting a physician. This book does not supply medical advice. Any application of the information herein is at the reader's own discretion and risk.

How would you like to receive free devotions in your inbox every weekday?

No fees. No catch.
No obligations.

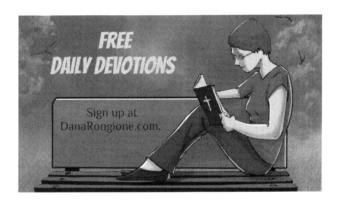

Sign up today at DanaRongione.com.

TABLE OF CONTENTS

INTRODUCTION

In the book of Nehemiah, the prophet by the same name was burdened by the Lord to take on a seemingly impossible task —to rebuild the wall of Jerusalem. Understand, this wall wasn't just weak or wobbly, it had completely crumbled and was lying in heaps of rubble. Nevertheless, where others saw brokenness, Nehemiah saw an opportunity and set out to do the impossible. Not only did he and the people rebuild the wall, but they did it in a mere fifty-two days despite the many obstacles hurled their way. Nehemiah had a burden, and he could not escape God's plan for him.

In the book, *Rise Up and Build: A Biblical Approach To Dealing With Anxiety and Depression*, I equate the building of the wall of Jerusalem to the building up of the walls we need to protect our spirits from rampant emotions and difficult circumstances. If you're dealing with anxiety and depression, I urge you to read that book too since it details all the elements necessary to fight off feelings of discouragement and worry. But for now, I want to talk with you about one of the most important—but often overlooked—things you can do for your emotional health. Using the story of Nehemiah, we'll uncover the secret to pushing past fear, exhaustion and depression and finding the strength to live the life God has always wanted us to have. Are you ready to get started?

STRENGTHEN FOR THE GOOD WORK

Then I told them of the hand of my God which was good upon me; as also the king's words that he had spoken unto me. And they said, Let us rise up and build. So they strengthened their hands for this good work. (Nehemiah 2:18)

I believe there's a lesson here for us. The first thing the people of Nehemiah's time did after declaring they would rise up and build was to strengthen their hands for the work. Sadly, this step is often skipped because of one of two reasons: (1) People don't understand the significance of taking care of the physical body in relation to dealing with emotional problems, or (2) People know but have no desire to embark on that part of the journey.

Yes, I'm talking about diet and exercise. Do you realize that most of the dis-

9

eases (physical, emotional and mental) we face today are linked to what we eat and our habits (or lack thereof) concerning exercise? It's true, and anxiety and depression are no exception. We are constantly feeding the very things that are draining our lives from us. And here's the crazy part: most of us refuse to change our eating and exercising. We reject the idea of strengthening our hands for the good work.

I'll discuss some of the excuses we make for clinging to our bad health habits in the next section, but for now, allow me to share with you another story from the Bible. In I Chronicles 21, King David sins against God and causes a plague to come upon the people of Israel. Repentant for his disobedience, David seeks to offer a sacrifice to God and plead for mercy. He goes to a man named Ornan and asks to buy a piece of his land on which he wants to offer the sacrifice to God. Ornan, being a good and gracious man, told David that he did not have to buy the land. Ornan would gladly give the land, the oxen for the sacrifice, the wood and whatever else David needed. But notice David's response: *And king David said to*

Ornan, Nay; but I will verily buy it for the full price: for I will not take that which is thine for the Lord, nor offer burnt offerings without cost (vs. 24).

David understood that a sacrifice that didn't cost him anything wasn't really a sacrifice at all. He understood the importance of going above and beyond for the Lord because God had certainly done that for him.

You're probably wondering what that has to do with our health and/or anxiety and depression. Allow me to explain. We are living sacrifices unto God (Romans 12:1), but too often we shy away from anything that's going to cost us something. The Bible tells us that the body is the temple of the Holy Ghost and that we should care for it, but we have a tendency to shrug off the conviction about our health because we know if we do what God is asking of us, it's going to cost us something. It will mean having to give up bad habits, junk food and some of our favorite treats. And sadly, as much as we love God, we obviously love our comfort foods more because we refuse to give them up.

The result is that we are destroying our bodies, and with them, our mental and emotional capabilities. We are unwilling to acknowledge that "garbage in; garbage out" is just as applicable in our physical and emotional health as it is anywhere else. We mistreat our bodies and fool ourselves into thinking that the only consequence is a little extra pudge. We have deluded ourselves and justified our poor health habits, and it has to stop!

I hope you are reading this book because you've reached the place of King David. I pray you've come to the point where you can say, "I know it's going to cost me something, but it's definitely worth it. I'm doing this for God, and I'm doing it for me!" If you're ready to be a living sacrifice fit for the Master's work, then let's get started, but first, let me ease your mind a bit.

Then he said unto them, Go your way, eat the fat, and drink the sweet, and send portions unto them for whom nothing is prepared: for this day is holy unto our Lord: neither be ye sorry; for the joy of the Lord is your strength. (Nehemiah 8:10)

Whoa! Did you catch that? Eat the fat. Drink the sweet. Fats and sweets? That's bad stuff, right? Not necessarily. What I'm going to share with you in this book has nothing to do with fad diets or severe calorie restriction. The trouble with fad diets is that they do not work and typically result in a vicious cycle of fatigue and discouragement. You start the diet with anticipation and excitement. For the first few weeks, the pounds drop off, and you gain momentum. Then, one day, your progress hits a brick wall. For the next week or so, despite your efforts, the scale refuses to budge, and before you know it, you've given up and gone back to your default eating habits. That is, until you've gained back all the weight that you had lost and then some. At that point, you realize you need to do something, and you begin the process all over again, only to be met with the same results. Let's face it, it's nearly impossible to maintain that type of program long-term. And that's what we need—a long-term solution. Remember, this isn't a quick fix. We're in this for the long haul, and that means making real changes that will last.

So, the first thing I want you to do is throw some words out of your vocabulary beginning with "diet." When we think "diet," we think of a short-term torture that we go through from time to time to lose weight. In order to achieve good health, we don't need to "diet." We need to change our relationship with food. You should also do away with concepts like "low fat," "low carb," and other such nonsense. It is not healthy to cut out food groups because our bodies need a proper balance, and we can't achieve that if we're cutting out life-giving nutrients that our bodies require. True nutrition is about eating the right foods in the proper proportions. That's it! It really is that simple, and in the next few chapters, I'll share with you how I have regained my health, lost weight, lowered my blood pressure, relieved emotional symptoms and much more while enjoying delicious, wholesome foods like ice cream, fried food and more. Yep, you read that right. Interested? Good!

Before we get to that, however, I want to make a couple more comments. This journey will require you to put aside all preconceived notions of how to eat right. This process is ultimately not about losing weight or shedding fat, though if done correctly, those things will follow suit. But, we cannot make the number on the scale our end goal. It's not about weight; it's about health. That being said, I want you to limit your time on the scale to once a week. Yep, that's it. There is no need to torture yourself every day by checking to see how much you've lost. Weight fluctuates based on water, salt intake and many other factors, so weighing yourself daily is a certain path to disappointment.

Personally, I use Saturday mornings to track my progress. First thing, I step on the scale and see where I am. No judgment. This is for information purposes only. Next, I measure my waist, one inch above my belly button. Lastly, I check my blood pressure. I keep a log of each of these figures so that I can view my progress over a period of time. Some weeks, the results are encouraging. Some weeks, not so much. But that's not the point. The biggest factor is how I am feeling overall. So, if you feel you must see numbers, please limit it to once each week and don't be disappointed if you don't see drastic changes.

Most fad diets bring about radical changes in a short amount of time. The problem is those changes are not sustainable, which is why people yo-yo so much in their weight. On the flip side, when we adopt healthy eating habits, the weight loss and changes in our physical features are slow but steady. That's what we want! That's the process that enabled me to make it through the Thanksgiving and Christmas holidays while continuing to lose weight. So, if you don't see big changes right away, don't get discouraged. Good things take time.

DISCLAIMER

Before I go any further, I am required to state that I am not a doctor, nutritionist, health coach or anything like that. I have no certifications or formal training to teach people how to eat and exercise, and that is not my ultimate goal. What I want to do is share with you what I've done (and am doing) to pursue my health goals and encourage you to make the changes necessary to improve your health. I urge you to consult your own physician or dietary specialist if you have questions or concerns.

Now, that we have all the legalities out of the way, let's talk about excuses.

EXCUSES

We, as humans, are skilled at coming up with excuses. Reading in the book of Genesis, we see how easily justifications for our poor decisions slip right off the tongue. When God confronted Adam and Eve about eating the forbidden fruit, Adam's response was, "Eve made me do it!" Seriously? But, alas, Eve's response wasn't any better. "The serpent tricked me!" Yes, it would appear that from the very beginning, we are prone to make excuses for poor behavior.

When it comes to taking care of our health, things are no different. I've heard them all. In fact, I've probably said them all. So, let's just go ahead and get these nasty little critters out of the way, shall we?

Excuse #1 - I would eat right, but it's too expensive.

I used this one for years, and being on a single income, I felt it was justified. But it's not. While I cannot necessarily afford to buy all organic foods, I can still use my money wisely and afford healthy food. An apple costs less than a candy bar. Water is cheaper than soda. We can afford it if we really want to. Plus, there are wonderful stores like Aldi and food surplus stores that carry high-quality foods at seriously discounted prices. Try it and see. Eating right is not as expensive as we think.

Excuse #2 - I would exercise, but I don't have the time.

The truth is we don't have the time NOT to exercise. Just a few minutes of motion floods our bodies with feel-good chemicals that are vital for boosting mood, improving focus and a whole host of other benefits. Ten minutes of exercise can produce thirty minutes or more of productivity.

Excuse #3 - I can't eat right because it's too complicated and takes too much time.

Been there, done that. But here's the thing—it doesn't have to be complicated. How difficult is it to grab an apple? Eating properly doesn't mean we have to become gourmet chefs (because if it did, I would be in BIG trouble). Keep it simple, and I'll tell you how in just a bit.

Excuse #4 - I can't exercise because I have injuries or I'm too tired.

Join the club! I think everyone these days is tired and has some form of injury or illness, but we can't use that as an excuse to lie around the house all day. We need to get moving, and believe it or not, exercise is exactly what we need to gain more energy and help our injuries. Our bodies weren't made to be sedentary. We've got to move it, move it!!!

Let's face it, we could spend all day listing the reasons why we can't eat right and exercise, but honestly, they don't hold water, do they? It's not that we can't but rather that we won't. So, let's change that thought pattern right now. We can do this because we can do all things through Christ who gives us strength (Philippians 4:13). This is something He wants for us. He desires for us to care for our bodies, so don't you think He'll give us the strength, motivation and passion to do just that? Of course He will. So, let's see where we need to begin.

DIET

What should go in your mouth? Let's make it very simple—if God made it, then let's eat it. If man made it, let's stay away. Empty your mind of everything you've been taught about carbs, fats and calories, and focus on the quality of the food. We all know that fruits and vegetables are good for us and contain life-giving nutrients, so eat lots of them. You can alter your entire way of eating by making little changes at a time. Trade out your soda for water. Try spreading avocado on your sandwich instead of mayonnaise. Make your meatloaf with oats instead of heavily processed breadcrumbs. Choose sunflower seeds instead of popcorn for your evening snack. Pretty soon those small changes turn into big results. And if you're really serious, you can even find healthy recipes that will have you feeling better and more fulfilled than ever.

What I'm saying is that you don't need special equipment or an expensive health program. There is no need to weigh your food or count your calories. If you're eating the right kind of food, everything else will fall into place. To get started, follow these simple steps:

1) Eat 4-6 small meals a day instead of 2-3 big ones. This is a huge component in healthy eating, especially on the emotional side of things. When we go long stretches without food, our blood sugar becomes unbalanced, which leads to mood swings and feelings of anxiety. Sometimes, the quickest way to rid ourselves of negative feelings is to eat something healthy. Remember, though, the key here is that they must be small meals. I had trouble with this when I first started because I was used to eating two or three BIG meals. I used to eat as much as my husband, I'm sorry to say. So, it took some adjustment to eating regularly, but I quickly found that I wasn't hungry, and my moods and energy levels were more stable throughout the day. Small meals include wraps, tortilla chips with salsa, pretzels and hummus, fruit, vegetables, a bowl of soup, a handful of nuts or seeds, etc.

2) Use a small plate instead of a large one. If there's room on our plate, we will fill it to the max, so when we use a small plate, we automatically limit our caloric intake without having to do any counting or measuring. A full plate tricks our brains into thinking that we're having more to eat, and our stomachs follow suit. Crazy, but it works!

3) Try to divide your plate into four sections. One quarter is for your protein (typically meat). One quarter is for your starch (rice, potatoes, bread, beans, etc.). One quarter is for non-starchy vegetables (greens, asparagus, broccoli, etc.). And the final quarter is for fruit. If you eat in these proportions, you'll find yourself satisfied without being full, and you'll slowly see more energy in your life.

4) Drink half your body weight in ounces of water per day. In other words, if you weigh 150 pounds, half of 150 is 75, which means you need to drink 75 ounces of water every day. Water is the only real energy drink, and if we want to be energized, there is no easier way than drinking our fill each and every day.

That's it! See, no big drama, but I guarantee you that if you follow the four steps above, you'll notice a definite change in your well-being—including physical, mental and emotional.

FOODS TO BE AVOIDED

While healthy eating is about much more than a list of dos and don'ts, there are a few "foods" that we should avoid at all costs if we are serious about wanting to improve our health. When it comes to these items, the word "food" is a relative term because, while these ingredients are found in many of the things we eat, they're not really foods.

The first of these health bashers is high fructose corn syrup. This harmful sweetener is in so much of our food, it's not even funny. In fact, an average American consumes sixty pounds of this stuff every year. Sixty pounds!!! From sodas to your favorite condiments, high fructose corn syrup makes its presence known by creating havoc in our bodies. How in the world this substance has been approved by the FDA, I'll never understand, but the truth is that many ailments and illnesses, such as obesity, cancer, dementia, heart disease and more, can be traced back to high fructose corn syrup. Personally, I found that HFCS was responsible for my chronic headaches and sinus issues, not to mention the spare tire around my middle that wouldn't go away no matter how many crunches I did. Once I gave up HFCS, these issues abated and my waistline decreased. We would be much better off to eat foods made with natural sweeteners such as honey, stevia or the sugars from fruits, so check your labels carefully, and if high fructose corn syrup is listed, skip it. You don't need it, and you'll be much better off without it.

Another thing to avoid is monosodium glutamate (MSG). This substance tops the charts of dangerous food additives. MSG is responsible for conditions such as neurological disorders, Alzheimer's, cardiac issues, kidney problems and much more. This additive alters hormones and messes with your brain chemistry, so obviously, if you're wanting to improve your health and emotions, this junk has got to go! Be warned. The food manufacturers have become quite devious and now disguise MSG by using other terms. When searching your labels, be on the lookout for ingredients like hydrolyzed vegetable protein, yeast extract, calcium caseinate, plant protein extract, and any textured proteins.

Similar to high fructose corn syrup, other artificial sweeteners have inundated our food supply. They promise fewer calories and a slimmer waistline, but what the creators fail to tell us is that these artificial sweeteners are like poison to our bodies. They are, as their name proudly proclaims, "artificial." In other words, they aren't real foods, and our bodies can't process them. So, when the marketers tout that their diet colas are better for you than regular colas, they're lying. Those diet drinks are just as bad, if not worse. Once again, we would do well to find products made with natural sugars such as sugar, honey, molasses, and the like.

Lastly, I want to mention something that isn't one specific item. Let's talk about processed foods. Processed foods are edible items that have been manufactured for longer shelf life. Typically, these "foods" are full of unpronounceable ingredients that read like a novel by J.R.R. Tolkein. Due to this processing, the food loses most of its nutritional value, and any goodness the food contained is replaced by excessive amounts of preservatives such as sodium. For the most part, any food in a box or can has been processed to some degree. To find out how good (or bad) a food is for you, check the ingredients. Wholesome foods should have fewer than ten ingredients (unless many of the ingredients are spices). Healthy foods should not contain any words that are a mile long and sound like another language. These are preservatives and fillers and should be avoided. Fortunately, many grocery stores are doing better about accommodating those of us who are looking for more nutritious foods and provide many options from which we can choose. While eating organic is best (if you can afford it), it is not necessary to see drastic improvement in your health. Simply paying attention to what's going into our bodies will go a long way toward healing them.

SIMPLE FOOD REPLACEMENTS

Getting on the path to healthy eating doesn't have to be drastic. Take your time and give your body a chance to get adjusted. I've discovered that the easiest way for me to shift into a new way of eating is to make small changes—or more specifically—exchanges. By exchanging a bad food for a healthier option, I'm improving my health one little step at a time, and the entire process seems much less daunting. Here are some easy substitutions you can make to ease your way into nutritious eating.

Use olive, grapeseed or coconut oil on your salad instead of dressing.

Use mashed avocado or hummus in place of mayonnaise.

Use oats instead of bread crumbs when making meatloaf.

Use brown rice pasta instead of white or wheat. Brown rice is naturally gluten free, and many people these days are having issues with gluten.

Use yogurt cheese instead of your regular cheeses. Many yogurt cheeses (despite the name) are lactose free and include a host of probiotics.

Use brown rice and brown sugar instead of white as it has been less processed.

Use ground turkey or chicken in place of beef.

Drink green tea instead of black. Black tea is horrible for inflammation!

Use sea salt instead of table salt.

Use olive oil, grapeseed oil, or coconut oil in place of vegetable, corn or sunflower oil.

Choose almond butter over peanut butter.

Eat organic when possible.

Use seeds (sunflower, pumpkin, flax, chia, etc.) in place of bacon bits and/or croutons.

MEAL PLAN; BE PREPARED

If we're honest, I think we'd all admit that we are compelled by convenience. Isn't it nice to eat out where someone else does the cooking and the cleanup? Oh yeah! The problem is that it's much easier to eat healthy and in the proper portion sizes at home than it is at a restaurant. And seriously, if we're thinking convenience, we're probably thinking fast food, which has nothing even resembling healthy to offer us.

If you want to succeed at eating healthy, the most important thing you can do is meal plan. Yes, I hear those groans. I know, it sounds awful. . .and tedious. . .and time-consuming. . .and. . . But here's the thing, it can be simple if you have the right tools and the proper approach.

You can do this with pen and paper, on the computer or even on your favorite electronic device (iPad, iPhone, etc.), but I've discovered that the easiest and most versatile method for me is using a pocket chart like the ones teachers use in their classrooms. (For an example, search Amazon for "pocket chart for classroom" and you'll see many options. Note: Make sure the chart you choose has at least seven pockets—one for each day of the week.)

Since this is my preferred method, I'll describe the process using the pocket chart, but it should be easy enough to figure out how to mimic the process elsewhere.

Step one is to make up little cards to use with your chart. I took 4x6 index cards and cut them into four pieces each. On each new card, I wrote down one of my favorite meals/snacks. I made cards until I couldn't think of anything else. When you're done with that, make one card for each day of the week and place those cards in the chart vertically.

For the next step, you need to determine how many meals each day you'll have. I have five, but you may prefer four or six. Do what works for you, your schedule and your family.

Now, it's simply a matter of sticking your meal/snack cards beside the day of the week you want to have them. There should be plenty of room for at least five cards per row, so you can fit all (or most if you have more meals) across the chart in order that you want to have them. Say, for example, that on Monday you wanted to have an energy bar when you woke up. Place that card in the pocket chart right after the word "Monday." After it, place the card stating your choice for Meal #2, then #3, and so on. You may find that, like me, you enjoy having the same thing for breakfast each day. That's fine. Put it in the first slot for the first day of the week and be done.

The convenience with this method is many-fold, but here are the two things I love most. First off, because the cards easily slip in and out of the pockets, rearranging meals is no big deal. If something happens and I need to switch tacos to Thursday instead of Tuesday, I just move the cards. It's that easy! Second, I place the chart on the refrigerator, so I rarely get asked, "What's for dinner?" My husband knows to look at the chart. Furthermore, if he's home before I am, he can start cooking because he knows the plan. For those of you with kids, the chart could benefit them as well when they come searching for a snack or are curious about the evening meal.

When the week is over, you can leave the chart the same, add some new items, or simply mix up the items already on the chart.

I keep all my extra cards in a Ziploc bag that stays with the chart, so it's always easy to add or subtract meals.

When it's time to make a grocery list, all I have to do is look down my meal plan chart and see what I need for each meal. The entire process can be done in a matter of minutes once you have everything set up.

And speaking of simple, if you want to make life even easier and don't mind eating the same foods regularly, you'll love the next section.

SIMPLIFY

I enjoy a variety of food, but I don't always enjoy having to decide what I want to eat from day to day. Sometimes, it seems like I take as long to decide what I'm having for lunch as it does to actually eat lunch. So, when I stumbled across a new idea, I decided to give it a try, and I'm so glad I did.

I still use my pocket chart for meal-planning, but the only meal I really plan for anymore is dinner. All of my other meals are repeats of the same thing.

For my first meal of the day, I have a homemade Almond Butter Energy bar. It is full of healthy fats, carbs and proteins and packs a powerful punch of sustaining energy to get me through the morning. These things are so yummy, it's almost like having dessert for breakfast.

Meal two alternates between falafel wraps and homemade soup and sandwiches. On Mondays, Wednesdays and Fridays, I have falafel wraps (see recipe in the last chapter). Tuesdays and Thursdays, I have veggie-filled soup (see recipe in the last chapter) and a grilled cheese sandwich, made with quality bread and yogurt cheese. A small bowl of fruit completes the meal.

My third meal consists of a homemade egg roll, fried in coconut oil. These veggie-stuffed delights are both delicious and filling. My husband makes up two dozen or so at a time, then places them in a bag in the freezer. When it's time for my snack, I get one out and drop it in the deep fryer. It couldn't be easier. . .or tastier! Occasionally, if I'm craving something lighter than an egg roll, I'll have pretzels and hummus, along with a piece of fruit.

My fourth meal of the day is dinner, which varies from day to day but always consists of healthy meal options like fish and veggies, shrimp stir fry, chicken fajitas, tacos, pasta and more.

Lastly, I finish my day with an avocado gelato/ice cream that is to die for. (Yes, I've included the recipe for you in the last chapter). It sounds strange, but I promise you, it's delicious. It tastes like ice cream. In fact, I've found that I prefer it to real ice cream because not only does it taste delicious, but it's healthy and leaves my stomach feeling relaxed and happy.

So, you see, with this plan in place, both meal planning and grocery shopping are a piece of cake. Plus, I don't have to spend time or energy wondering what I'm going to eat at every meal. I already know. The best part is that once I finally got everything adjusted perfectly, I found myself in a slight calorie deficit, which means that I'm losing weight without ever having to weigh or count anything. And because I'm adhering to these good habits regularly, I can even treat myself to something special now and then and never notice a change in my health or weight.

You may not like the idea of eating the same foods every day, and that's fine. The important thing is that you make a plan and be prepared. Keep healthy, convenient foods on hand so you'll never find yourself reaching for the cookie jar simply because it's easy. If necessary, keep healthy options in the car, your purse or briefcase and wherever else you may find yourself giving in to the temptation of convenience. Chances are if you have the proper food on hand, you'll eat that instead of spending the time or money to get something else.

TIPS AND TIMESAVERS

One of the biggest complaints people have about eating healthy is that it is too costly and time-consuming. While it does take a bit more time to shop for and prepare your own meals, it is actually much more affordable than eating out, not to mention, better for your health. Still, to aid you in your efforts, here are a few tips and timesavers I've found especially profitable.

First off, when purchasing your food, don't overlook bargain food stores and farmer's markets. Many of these places offer high quality foods at discounted prices. For example, a nearby farmer's market provides what I need for produce, eggs and dairy. A discount food store is within thirty miles of my house, and it has proven to be a wonderful discovery. Not only are their prices phenomenal, but they offer many organic and high-quality foods that I couldn't afford to purchase elsewhere. As far as local supermarkets go, if you have an Aldi near you, they also provide many nutritious options at very reasonable prices. Eating right doesn't require you to do all your shopping at expensive health food boutiques. Look around your area, and find places that offer high-quality foods at good prices.

While we're discussing shopping, here's another time and money-saving tip. Did you know that you can purchase a fully-cooked rotisserie chicken for the exact same price as a raw chicken? Yes, I'm serious! Talk about easy. You don't even have to cook the thing. We love this option as it makes meal planning and preparation a cinch. Basically, take the bird home and debone it. Put the bones aside (we'll talk about them in just a moment) and place the meat in a Ziploc bag. There's only two of us, so we typically get about three to four meals out of that one bird. When it's dinner time, we get out what we need of the meat and add it to whatever else our meal involves, whether it be fajitas or stir fry. Make the mess once; eat off that meat for an entire week. I love it! You can follow a similar method when fixing a bigger roast. Cook it, debone it (if it has bones), then plan several meals around that meat. Easy, peasy!

Now, let's talk about those bones. In the last chapter, I'll give you a recipe for making your own bone broth. Bone broth has a variety of health benefits, and making your own is both cost-efficient and nutritious because you know exactly what's in it. Typically, we freeze the bones in a baggie until we have two chickens worth. Then, we make up a large batch of broth. Once the broth has cooled, we divide it up into mason jars. We place one in the refrigerator and the others in the freezer for later use. When we're ready to make a soup or need a broth base for one of our favorite recipes, we have plenty of healthy options on hand. Make once; use for several occasions to come.

As you can see, I'm a huge fan of easy. The truth is, I don't like to cook. It is not a passion of mine at all, but it must be done. So, I try to make things as simple as possible. If I have to go through the time and effort of making something, I do my best to make much more than we need and freeze the leftovers for easy meals at a later time. For example, dinner tonight will be chili. Did I make chili today? Nope! I made it a few weeks ago, and placed two large containers of "extras" in the freezer. This morning, I got one of the containers out of the freezer and set it in the sink to thaw. At dinner time, I'll dump the chili into a saucepan and heat. That's it! I do the same thing with soups, meatloaves, burgers, muffins and much more. I've learned it doesn't really take more time or effort to make a bigger portion of food, but it certainly saves a lot of time and effort the next occasion (or two) we have that meal. If you can make extra and freeze the leftovers, I encourage you to do so. You'll thank yourself later!

EXPECT DETOX

I cannot, in good conscience, urge you to change your eating habits without mentioning the process of detoxification. When you start filling your body with healthy foods, it begins to clean itself out. Basically, the body tries to rid itself of all the built-up toxins by pulling them out "into the open" so that it can use the body's natural processes of elimination. The toxins that have been hiding in fat stores are now floating in the body and can make you feel miserable. Some common symptoms of detoxification are severe headache, skin breakouts, body odor, stomachache, clogged sinuses, fever, body aches, fatigue, and irritability. Sounds like fun, huh? When the symptoms first appear, it's tempting to stop the healthy eating and go back to your old ways, but please don't! Follow through. The symptoms will pass as your body eliminates the unhealthy elements. To ease the process, drink more water. The more water you drink, the quicker and easier it is for your body to eliminate the toxins.

You're probably wondering why you would want to put yourself through all that. I can't explain to you how much better you'll feel once your system has been cleaned out. Not only will the cleansing symptoms disappear, but I guarantee you'll notice other areas of improvement in your well-being. By unclogging your body, you allow it to operate more effectively and efficiently. This will be evident in reduced sickness, increased energy levels, improved mood, and a host of other areas.

Remember, what good is a sacrifice if it doesn't cost us anything? Yes, it will be uncomfortable for a little while (typically a week or so), but just think how much better you'll look and feel afterward. I promise you it's worth it. Just hang tough, and keep eating the right things!

EXERCISE

I hear the groans already. Don't worry. This chapter will be relatively painless, but it is a necessary topic. We live in a society of sitters. We sit at the desk. We sit on the sofa. We sit on the pew. We sit and sit and sit all day long. Is it any wonder the majority of our population is suffering from obesity and many other diseases that could be prevented if we would get off our—ahem, "seats"— and move? We were not made to be sedentary all day. I guarantee you there were no easy chairs in the Garden of Eden. We were made to move, and when we fail to do that, our bodies suffer.

Unfortunately, we have a tendency to make our lack of exercise a joke. We quote the first part of I Timothy 4:8, which reads, *For bodily exercise profiteth little*, and use it as a Biblical proof text that exercise is not important when we know that's not what God is saying. We understand that exercise is important; we're just too lazy to do it. (Sorry, but the truth hurts!)

Now, I will be the first to admit that the thought of going to the gym makes me cringe. I do not like the gym. I don't like the equipment. I don't like the setting. I don't like the ambience. And honestly, I don't particularly like a lot of the people. I feel judged, inferior and clumsy in the presence of many gym rats. So, I avoid the gym as much as possible, but that doesn't mean I have an excuse not to move my body.

I'm going to let you in on a little secret. I have discovered the best exercise ever. Are you ready for this? The best exercise is any movement that you will do regularly. Yep, I'm serious. Maybe it's playing with the dog in the backyard or throwing a frisbee with your kids. Perhaps, like me, you enjoy walking or hiking. Maybe you're a real daredevil and prefer activities like rock climbing or ninja training. Whatever it is, find some form of movement that you enjoy doing, and do it daily if possible. You don't have to run five miles a day or climb Mount Everest to improve your health. You would be amazed at how much better you'll feel if you'll take a 10-minute walk as part of your lunch break every day. Little changes can add up to big results.

When I first began going on morning prayer walks, I struggled to hobble along for a mile. This morning, I walked three-and-a-quarter miles in under one hour, and my day has been brighter and more productive because of it. Plus, by combining my prayer with my exercise, I free up more time for other things, and honestly, my prayer walks are when I feel the closest to the Lord. I cherish that activity each and every day (weather permitting, of course).

So, you see, it doesn't have to be complicated or time-consuming. Find something you enjoy doing and do it. Do it with a friend. Work out with your family. Spend that activity time with the Lord. Whatever. There are no rules except this—Move it!

EXERCISING WITHOUT EQUIPMENT

Contrary to popular opinion, you don't need special equipment to get a complete workout. In fact, you can get a full workout by doing bodyweight exercises in which you don't need any equipment at all. The key is to focus on working every muscle in the body evenly. In other words, you don't want to do 100 pushups and never do any leg work. (By the way, if you can do 100 pushups, you probably don't need my help.)

Some popular bodyweight exercises include pushups, sit ups, pull ups (if you have a bar or beam somewhere that will hold your weight—just a side note, a towel bar will not work, and I would prefer not to say how I know this), squats, lunges, calf raises, wall sits, planks, and dips (can be done with two chairs or small tables). Add some cardio work like jumping jacks or running in place, and you have a complete workout that can be done in no time and requires no special or costly equipment.

If you would like to purchase some equipment but are short on room and cash, I would advise you pick up a chin-up bar and two or three different length resistance bands. That's it! Once again, you can get a very effective workout with just these few items. Chin-up bars can be purchased for around $10, and resistance bands are generally $5-$10 each, depending on the size and quality. I personally have the bar and three different resistance bands, although I've found I can get by with the longest and shortest ones.

If you're unsure how to use resistance bands or are unfamiliar with the myriad of exercises you can do with them, I strongly suggest you do a quick online search. Just type in "resistance band exercises" or "resistance band workout." The results will astound you. The thing I love about resistance bands is they're lightweight and easy to use. I can travel with them. I can carry them from room to room or even outside if the weather is nice. They are safe and effective, and I get the advantage of working with weight without the fear of dropping a ten-pound dumbbell on my foot.

For a fun bodyweight exercise routine, search YouTube for "The Scientific 7-Minute Workout." This brief workout targets the entire body. I don't do it every morning, but I try to add it into my weekly run of routines. It's quick, but I promise you, you'll feel a difference, and don't be surprised if you find your body aching for the first few days. (Trust me, that's a good sign.) The video contains a couple of exercises that I can't do because of physical issues, so I substitute in movements I can do. What I love about this particular video is that it combines strength training with cardio, and it keeps track of time, so I don't have to. I hope you'll enjoy it as well.

Speaking of injuries, let's talk about that next.

EXERCISING WITH INJURIES

Our human tendency is to avoid pain at all cost. So when an injury flares up, our first instinct is to "baby" it and avoid doing anything that might cause it more pain. Well, here's a newsflash, when you start exercising, you will experience pain, especially if you have an injury. The first few weeks of exercising with my bursitis and arthritis were torturous, but I'm so glad I followed through. You see, even though our bodies are experiencing pain, that doesn't necessarily mean that what we're doing is a bad thing. It just means that the part of the body that is injured isn't happy. Chances are, however, that exercise is exactly what it needs. Remember, to check with your doctor before starting any exercise program to make sure the movements won't cause further damage.

The key to exercising with an injury is to work yourself into it. You're most likely not going to be able to do a full thirty-minute workout the first time. That's okay. You don't have to. If you can only do five minutes, then do five minutes. Make an effort to repeat that five minute workout every other day for a week. After that, see if you can increase it to ten minutes. Then, see if you can do ten minutes every day instead of every other day. You see how it works? You have to push yourself some, but if you push too hard, your body will push right back, and you'll find yourself in a place you don't want to be. Take it easy. Take it slow. But be determined.

By far, my favorite exercise is walking. It's easy to do. It requires little time and no equipment except a decent pair of shoes. But I think what I love most about walking is that it benefits my mind and spirit as much as it does my body. I don't know what it is about walking, but it's soothing and energizing all at the same time. When I walk, I can literally feel my muscles unwinding and un-kinking. At the same time, my mind becomes more focused and my spirit feels more free. Mind you, the kind of walking of which I'm speaking is not done on a treadmill or in laps around a yard or gym, although each of those types of walking certainly has health benefits. Rather, the type of walking of which I'm speaking is trail walking, you know, where you get on a trail (paved or not) and just walk. The best trails are those that are surrounded by nature. Fortunately, there is just such a trail right down the road from my house.

Walking is a simple enough exercise that it can be completed while I talk to God. Yes, if you've never tried prayer walking, you are truly missing out. Prayer walking, as its name implies, is simply talking and listening to God while you walk, making the walk a benefit for the spiritual nature as well as the physical, mental and emotional. Walking al-lows me to sort things out, both with myself and with God. It allows me to clear my head and balance my emotions. And it gives me time to get alone with God, to pour out my heart to Him, to seek His counsel and to rest in His love. It is a truly joyous time that I treasure.

As one who suffers from both arthritis and bursitis, I can attest to the pain-relieving properties of a good walk. The fluid movement of walking helps to lubricate and loosen the joints of the body, thus enabling better range of motion and a reduction in pain and swelling. There is no right or wrong way to walk, but I have found that I receive the most benefit when I walk briskly while allowing my arms to hang and swing freely. If you find that you're at a point where brisk walking is beyond you, that's fine. Start slowly. A slow walk is better than no walk at all.

Whether you're looking to lose weight, improve your health, balance your emotions, increase your mental focus or spend time with God, walking can help. You don't have to walk long or fast; just walk. Before long, you'll be able to walk farther and faster than you ever dreamed possible. But more than that, you'll be amazed to discover that you long to walk. You'll start to crave it. And when that happens, you can take great comfort in the realization that you've implemented a new healthy habit into your life.

After that, I suggest adding a gentle stretching routine like pilates. Your muscles are tired and sore, and chances are, the injured area has grown weak and the muscles have drawn up. Before you begin working the muscles, it's important to stretch them out. Spend a few minutes preparing your muscles for your workout. If you're not sure about the best stretches for your body, I recommend YouTube. You can find all kinds of stretching recommendations. Some of the videos are short while others are long. Find what works for you.

If, after several weeks of stretching and walking, you feel like you can do more, start off with resistance band workouts. This makes it easy to adjust the weight if you feel you've taken on too much. The important thing to remember is to keep your movements smooth and gentle. Pay attention to your body. Learn to distinguish between the pain of unfamiliar use and the pain of true in-

jury.   And above all, work your way into it.
Slow and steady wins the race!

REST

Lastly, when discussing how to take care of our physical bodies, we can't ignore the importance of rest. Yes, I know, you're busy. I know you have a lot to do and little time to do it. I understand that when you do take time out to rest, you feel lazy and have this weird assumption that everyone else is accusing you of being lazy as well. But rest is not an option; it's a necessity. Even God Himself set aside a time to rest. What makes us think we can buzz along on all cylinders and never take a break? It doesn't work. Our bodies demand rest, and if your body is anything like mine, it will stop and drop whether I want it to or not, so I've found it's better to stop and take a break before my body makes me stop.

Now, you may be wondering, how much rest do we really need? Honestly, that all depends on the individual. If my husband sleeps six hours a night, he does great. As for me, my body needs around nine or ten hours. Yep, you read that right—nine or ten hours, and no, I'm not related to Rip Van Winkle. So, you know what I do? I sleep ten hours per night and get more done while I'm awake because I'm not spending all day yawning and trying to keep myself from dozing off. And if, by chance, I do still feel tired, I take a short rest around mid-day. I'm not much of a napper, so I seldom sleep during the day, but taking a few minutes to close my eyes and rest my body does wonders to refresh my mind and spirit.

Here's the key to finding out how much sleep you need: go to bed and wake up at the same time every day. My bedtime is 8:30, and I do my very best to be in bed by that time every night. The reason I do that is because I'm most productive in the morning and least productive in the evening, so I have adjusted my bedtime to suit my schedule. By going to bed at the same time every night, my body automatically wakes itself up at the right time in the morning, typically around 6:00. I don't need to be jarred awake by an alarm clock. I don't have to get up before my body is fully rested. My body does the work, and I reap the benefits. You can do the same. Start by setting your alarm clock for the time you need to get up (until your body is trained to wake up on its own, you'll need to use the alarm clock). If you currently do not wake up before your alarm, try going to bed a half hour earlier each night for the next couple of weeks. If you're still not waking up before your alarm, go to bed a half hour earlier still. Keep pushing your bedtime back every couple of weeks until you consistently wake up before your alarm. This will give you a good indication of how much sleep your body needs. Once you've determined your body's rest requirements, try to meet that quota as much as you can. This makes a huge difference in energy levels and overall mood.

RECIPES

OMELET MUFFINS

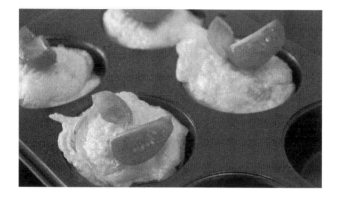

What if you could have the tastiness of bacon and eggs in a convenient package that could be eaten in the car on the way to work? Now, you can. Bacon and eggs, meet muffins! Who said convenient foods couldn't be good for you?

INGREDIENTS:

8 eggs

8 ounces crumbled cooked ham, sausage or bacon (nitrite and nitrate-free)

1 cup diced bell pepper

1 cup diced onion

¼ teaspoon salt

⅛ teaspoon ground black pepper

2 tablespoons milk

1 cup mushrooms (optional)

1 cup cherry tomatoes (optional)

Additional seasonings (optional) - Personally, I love rosemary in my eggs!

PROCESS:

Preheat oven to 350°F. Grease 8 muffin cups or line with paper liners.

Beat eggs together in a large bowl. Mix meat choice, bell pepper, onion, salt, black pepper, and milk into the beaten eggs. Pour egg mixture evenly into prepared muffin cups.

Bake in the preheated oven until muffins are set in the middle, 18 to 20 minutes.

PROTEIN PANCAKES

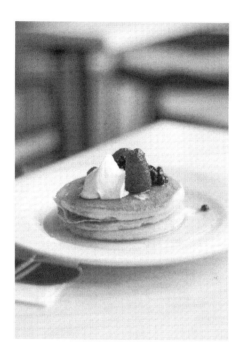

If you love pancakes but don't want to be
weighed down by heavy starches, you'll love
these four-ingredient pancakes.
So easy yet so tasty.

INGREDIENTS:
1 large banana
2 eggs
⅛ teaspoon baking powder (optional but recommended)
2 tablespoons vanilla whey protein powder (optional; you can also add a touch of vanilla extract instead)

PROCESS:
Place a medium skillet over medium heat on the stove, and let it heat up while you prepare the pancakes. It's ready when water dropped into the pan sizzles.
To prepare the pancakes, mash the banana well with a fork.
Add the eggs, baking powder, and protein powder (if using) and whisk until well combined. (You can use a mixer if that works better for you.)
Drop some olive oil or coconut oil into the pan and spread around before adding in 2-3 tablespoons of the pancake mixture.
Let the pancakes cook for 25-30 seconds before flipping and letting the other side cook for the same amount of time. (You'll

know they're ready to flip when you see
bubbles forming on the top.)
Remove to a plate and serve with nut butter,
butter, fruit, or whatever you'd like! (I love
butter, fruit and honey. Yum!)

HEALTHY EGG ROLLS

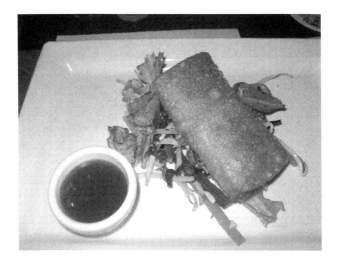

Having trouble getting in enough veggies? What if you could have a tasty, low-calorie snack that is packed full of nutritious vegetables? These egg rolls are delicious and filling, making them the perfect mid-afternoon snack.

INGREDIENTS:
12 egg roll wrappers
½-1 lb ground pork, chicken or beef, or chopped shrimp
2 teaspoons chopped fresh ginger
2 garlic cloves, minced
1 teaspoon salt
1 teaspoon sugar
¼ cup soy sauce
1 teaspoon sesame oil
1 (16 ounce) bag of shredded cabbage and carrot coleslaw mix
Two handfuls of bean sprouts
4 green onions, sliced
1 egg, beaten (optional)
1 teaspoon water
Coconut oil (for frying)

PROCESS:
Brown the meat with ginger and garlic in pan; drain any grease.
Mix salt, sugar, soy sauce and sesame oil. Add to the meat and mix well.
In large bowl, combine cabbage mix, bean sprouts and green onions.
Pour hot meat over vegetables and stir well. Let cool slightly.

Lay wrap in front of you so that it looks like a diamond.

Place 3 tablespoons of filling in center of egg roll wrapper.

Fold bottom point up over filling and roll once.

Fold in right and left points.

Brush beaten egg on top point. (This step is optional. You can use a little water instead.) Finish rolling.

Set aside and repeat with remaining filling.

Heat 2-3 inches oil in large frying pan to very hot (350°F), or you can use a deep fryer if you have one.

Fry a few egg rolls in pan at a time, 2-3 minutes per side.

Drain on paper towels.

Serve hot.

NOTES:
Because this is a longer process and it's hard to eat this many egg rolls at once, you can prepare them (but do not cook), lay them on a cookie sheet and place them in the freezer. Once the egg rolls are frozen, place them in freezer bags and store them in the freezer until you're ready for them.

When you're ready for a snack, get out the number of egg rolls you desire and allow them to thaw for 15 to 20 minutes, then fry.

BONE BROTH

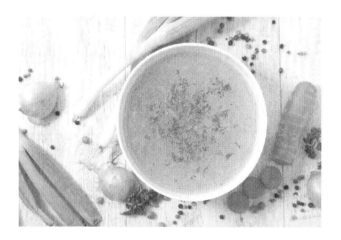

In case you haven't heard, bone broth is one of the healthiest foods on the planet. It is full of so many vitamins and nutrients that our bodies need. And if you suffer from any joint issues, you'll love the benefits you can gain from consuming bone broth regularly. While it is a timely process, it is so simple!

INGREDIENTS:
4 lbs bones (beef, chicken, turkey, pork)
12 cups water
2 tablespoons apple cider vinegar
1 medium onion, roughly diced
1 ½ cups chopped carrots
1 ½ cups chopped celery
3 bay leaves
3-5 sprigs fresh rosemary
6 cloves garlic
1 teaspoon black pepper

PROCESS:
Throw all the ingredients into your crockpot and set it on medium to high. Allow to cook and simmer for 24 to 48 hours, adding water as needed. Once it's done, strain the broth into a container (or containers) and place it (them) in the refrigerator or freezer, depending on how soon you intend to use it. (We typically have three or four jars of broth ready and waiting for making delicious soups.)

SUPERFOOD CHICKEN STEW

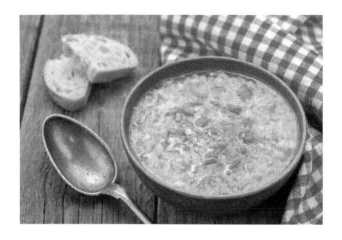

Remember that nutritious bone broth we made, well, here's a perfect place to use it. This hearty stew is packed full of superfoods. Serve alone or with a side of bread or a grilled cheese sandwich.

INGREDIENTS:
4 medium carrots, chopped
¼ cup chopped onion
½ cup dry wild rice
4 cups fresh spinach, tightly packed
½ lb. mushrooms
½ lb. broccoli
2 cloves garlic, minced
4 chicken breast fillets, add raw chicken cut into 2" chunks (see note below)
4 cups chicken broth
1(28 oz.) can diced tomatoes, with juice
1 (15 oz.) can kidney beans

PROCESS:
Add ingredients to the slow cooker in the same order as above. For example, place carrots on the bottom, followed by rice, spinach, mushrooms, broccoli, garlic, chicken, broth, tomatoes and lastly beans. Cover and cook on low 6-8 hours.

NOTES:
If you don't like messing with raw chicken or prefer to not have to pay for chicken breasts, you can use a fully-cooked rotisserie chicken instead. Simply wait to add the

chicken until about 30 minutes before you plan to serve the soup.

FALAFEL WRAPS

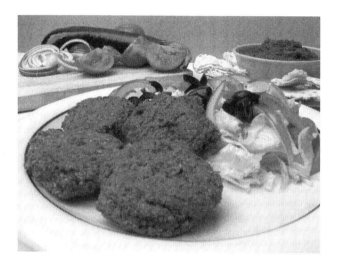

As crazy as it sounds, these little vegetarian delights have become one of my favorite meals. They're sustaining yet sit so lightly on the stomach. The process seems a little daunting at first, but you can make dozens of falafels at a time and place them in the freezer to use as needed. Overall, it's a huge time-saver and perfect for those times you want something light yet filling.

INGREDIENTS:
16-oz dried chickpeas
2 cloves garlic, lightly crushed
½ onion, quartered
1 teaspoon ground coriander
1 tablespoon ground cumin
1 teaspoon cayenne, or to taste
½ cup chopped fresh parsley or cilantro
1 teaspoon salt
½ teaspoon freshly ground black pepper
½ teaspoon baking soda
1 tablespoon freshly squeezed lemon juice
Coconut oil, for deep-frying

PROCESS:
Put beans in a large bowl and cover with water by 3 to 4 inches—they will triple in volume as they soak. Soak for 24 hours, checking once or twice to see if you need to add water to keep the beans covered. Drain beans well and transfer to a food processor with all the remaining ingredients except the oil; pulse until minced but not puréed; add water tablespoon by tablespoon if necessary to allow the machine to do its work, but keep the mixture as dry as possible. (If your moisture is too wet to keep

shape, add a touch of flour.) Taste and adjust seasoning, adding more salt, pepper, cayenne or a little more lemon juice as needed.

Put at least 2 to 3 inches of oil (more is better) in a large deep saucepan (or use a deep fryer). Turn heat to medium high and heat oil to about 350°F.

Scoop out heaping tablespoons of the mixture and shape it into balls or small patties. (The mixture should be dry enough that it doesn't stick to your fingers.) Fry in batches, without crowding, until nicely browned, turning as necessary; total cooking time per batch will be less than 5 minutes. Serve hot or at room temperature.

NOTE:

Falafels can be eaten on their own or within a bigger meal. Our favorite way to eat them is in a wrap. Spread hummus and/or avocado on a flour tortilla. Fill the tortilla with your favorite veggies (bell peppers, onions, celery, olives, mushrooms, tomatoes, spinach, etc.). Crumble the falafel on top of the veggies and fold the tortilla closed. That's it! Serve with chips and salsa, homemade fries or a side vegetable.

STUFFED PEPPERS

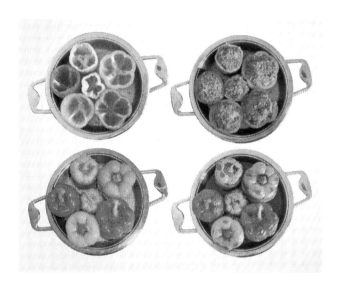

When I eat this meal, it reminds me of pasta with a twist. Not only is it pleasing to the taste buds, but it's actually good for you too. Win, win!

INGREDIENTS:
4 large bell peppers
1 lb of ground beef or turkey (white meat is healthier, just saying)
½ small onion (chopped)
1 cup of <u>cooked</u> brown rice
1 teaspoon salt
⅛ teaspoon garlic salt
1 tablespoon Italian seasoning (optional)
1 can tomato sauce (15 oz)
1-1½ cup shredded mozzarella or yogurt cheese

PROCESS:
Preheat oven to 350°F.
Cut a circle around the top of the pepper and remove it (making a lid).
Cut out seeds and membranes.
Cook in boiling water for 5-7 minutes.
Drain.
While peppers are boiling, brown the ground beef (or turkey) until cooked through.
Add in onion and cook until softened.
Drain and return to the skillet.
Mix in ¼-1/3 cup of cheese.

Add the rice, salt, garlic salt and 1 cup of
tomato sauce to the meat. Cook until all is
hot.
Spoon the meat mixture into the peppers.
Stand upright in a small baking dish.
Pour the remaining sauce over the tops of
the peppers.
Cover with foil and bake for 45 min.
Uncover and sprinkle with cheese.
Bake until cheese is melted.

RISE UP AND BUILD

SALMON PATTIES

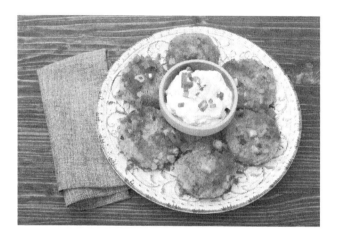

For those of you who know the health benefits of seafood but really aren't a huge fan of the taste, here's a great way to eat that fish and love it too.

INGREDIENTS:

14.75 oz. can salmon

½ medium onion, chopped

½ cup breadcrumbs, crackers or flour

¼ cup chopped parsley (optional)

2 eggs, beaten

2 tablespoons unsalted butter

3 tablespoons olive oil

salt

pepper

PROCESS:

Sauté onions in 1 TBS olive oil until cooked through but not brown.

Drain liquid from the salmon and be sure to remove all the bones.

Combine salmon, sautéed onion, breadcrumbs, eggs, salt, and pepper.

Form mixture into patties.

Melt butter and oil in a pan.

Brown salmon patties on both sides (about 4-5 minutes per side).

Place cooked patties on a paper towel to absorb excess oil.

NOTE:
While I do enjoy salmon, the process of dealing with the bones irritates and annoys me, so I choose to make this recipe with tuna instead. It works exactly the same except you don't have to deal with bones. I typically make mine with coconut flour (rather than bread crumbs) as the binder and serve the patties over a fresh salad. Yummy, and surprisingly filling!

EASY LASAGNA TOSS

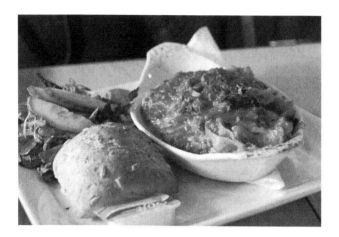

I love lasagna, but I do not enjoy the time that it takes to prepare. With this beauty of a recipe, you can have tantalizing pasta on the table in less than an hour. Oh yeah!

INGREDIENTS:
1 lb. lean ground beef or turkey
1 jar (24 oz.) Pasta Sauce
1 2/3 cups water
2 bell peppers, chopped
1 onion, chopped
3 cloves garlic, minced
12 brown rice lasagna noodles, each broken into smaller pieces
1 cup mozzarella or yogurt cheese

PROCESS:
Brown meat in large saucepan; drain.
Add pasta sauce, water, peppers, onion and cloves; mix well. Bring to boil.
Stir in noodles; cover.
Cook on medium-low heat 30 minutes or until noodles are tender, stirring occasionally. Remove from heat. Sprinkle with cheese; cover. Let stand 5 min. or until cheese is melted.
Serve with a side of healthy greens or tossed salad.

CROCKPOT TERIYAKI CHICKEN

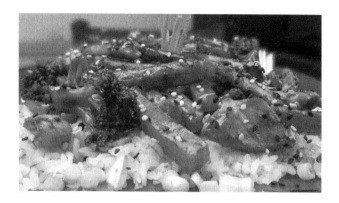

Who doesn't love takeout? Now, you can save some money and make your own. I promise it's easy and tastes like it came from a restaurant. Best of all, you can combine it with a few of the egg rolls you made earlier and make it a complete feast.

INGREDIENTS:

1 pound diced chicken (see note below)
½ cup teriyaki sauce
1 cup chicken broth (see note below)
1/3 cup brown sugar
3 cloves garlic minced
1 bag stir-fry veggies (fresh or frozen)

PROCESS:

Combine chicken broth, teriyaki sauce, brown sugar and garlic cloves in large bowl. Add chicken and veggies to sauce, and toss to combine.

Pour chicken and veggie mixture into crock-pot.

Cook on low 4-6 hours, or until chicken is cooked through.

Serve over cooked brown rice and spoon extra sauce if desired

NOTE:

* You can use the rotisserie chicken here as well. Stir it into the crockpot 30 minutes before you serve the meal. Overall cook time can be reduced to 2-4 hours because you're not having to cook the chicken.

** Here's another wonderful use for your homemade bone broth.

MEATLOAF

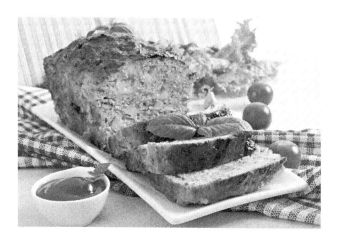

If you have a little more time to fix dinner
and find yourself in the mood for some home
cooking, you'll enjoy this healthy version of a
comfort food classic. The only bad part is
that it's so delicious, you'll want to have
seconds and thirds and. . .

INGREDIENTS:
2 teaspoons olive oil
1 medium onion, finely chopped
1 cup chopped carrot
½ cup chopped celery
¼ cup chopped green onion
¼ cup chopped mushrooms
2 cloves garlic, minced
1/8 teaspoon thyme
1 egg
1 cup oats
½ cup ketchup (optional)
¼ teaspoon salt
1 lb ground turkey
½ lb ground beef

PROCESS:
Preheat oven to 375°F. Spray an 8"x4" loaf
pan with vegetable cooking spray. Set aside.
In a large nonstick skillet, heat oil over
medium-high heat. Add vegetables, garlic,
and thyme. Cook, stirring until vegetables
began to soften, about five minutes. Transfer
to a plate and cool slightly.
In a large bowl, combine the egg whites,
oats, ketchup (if using), and salt. Add turkey
and beef; mix until blended. Add vegetable

mixture, and mix well. Press into the prepared pan.
Bake for 45 to 55 minutes. Let stand for 10 minutes. Cut into slices and serve.

NOTE:
Meatloaf slices can be placed in individual sealed bags and frozen for later use.

CHICKEN ENCHILADAS

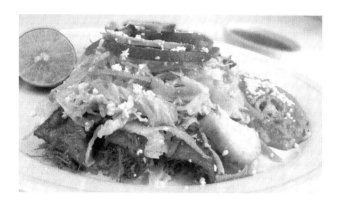

Here's an interesting twist on a Mexican classic. If you like enchiladas, I think you'll enjoy this simple dinner plan.

INGREDIENTS:
2 teaspoon olive oil
1 bell pepper
1 onion
1 can black beans, drained
1 tablespoon cumin
1 tablespoon garlic
1-2 tsp chili powder
½-1 small can enchilada sauce
4-6 oz cooked chicken(see note)
Flour tortillas
Shredded cheese

PROCESS:
Preheat oven to 350°F.
Heat the oil in a medium pan.
Add pepper and onion. Sauté until nearly soft.
Add black beans, seasoning and enchilada sauce. Allow to simmer for 5 minutes.
Add chicken until the mixture is thick and no longer soggy and cook for another 5 minutes.
Lay tortillas out on cookie sheet.
Spoon chicken mixture into one half of each tortilla, then fold the tortilla, making it like a taco.

Sprinkle cheese on top.

Bake in the oven approximately 5 minutes or until the cheese is melted.

Serve immediately. This goes well with a side of greens, or my favorite is to top the enchilada with a salad of lettuce, tomatoes, peppers, onion, celery, etc. The cool, crispy salad on top of the warm tortilla blend is heavenly!

NOTE:

*Feel free to use your rotisserie chicken.

**You can opt to roll your tortillas into a traditional enchilada shape and place them side by side in a baking dish. Sprinkle cheese over the entire thing and bake. For me, this is more time-consuming, so I do it the easy way. You choose!

CHOCOLATE AVOCADO GELATO/ICE CREAM

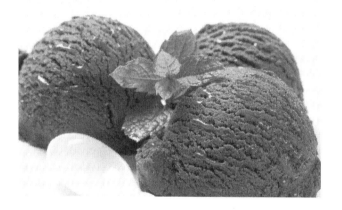

Oh my goodness! This is my favorite recipe EVER!!!! This girl loves chocolate, and I'm quite a big fan of ice cream too, so when I discovered this gem, I was so happy. To this day, I still prefer it over regular ice cream, and the best part of all is, not only is it not bad for you, it's actually good for you. Can I get an "Amen"?

INGREDIENTS:
1 avocado, peeled and pitted
½ cup canned coconut milk (you can also use almond, hemp or rice milk if you want)
3 tablespoon unsweetened cocoa powder
¼-½ cup maple syrup or honey (depends on how sweet you like it)
½ teaspoon vanilla extract
Dash of salt
Mini chocolate chips (optional)

PROCESS:
Add the avocado and coconut milk to a food processor or blender and pulse together. Add the remaining ingredients and blend for about 2 minutes until smooth and incorporated, scraping down the bowl once. Pour into a container and freeze, covered, until frozen solid (usually about 4-6 hours). You may want to let the ice cream sit on the counter and soften a bit before trying to serve. It can get quite stiff.
Enjoy with your favorite toppings like nuts, coconut, fruit, etc.

NOTE:
This is a very flexible recipe and can be adapted to fit your taste. You can add other flavors like peanut butter, mint extract, or fruit. You can also dump in other ingredients like nuts and such. The possibilities are endless. Just remember to keep it healthy. That's the best part about this guilt-free dessert!

ENERGY BALLS

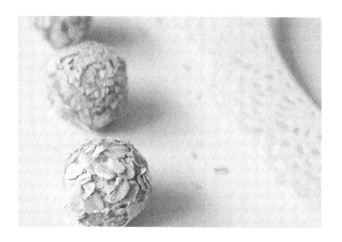

I'm sorry, but there are very few store-bought protein bars that I actually enjoy. Most of them taste like the cardboard boxes they're sold in. Yuck! These little balls, however, have a different story to tell, and they're so quick and easy to make.

INGREDIENTS:

1 cup (dry) oats

2/3 cup toasted coconut flakes

½ cup peanut butter

½ cup ground flax, sunflower or pumpkin seeds

½ cup dark chocolate chips

1/3 cup honey or agave nectar

1 tablespoon chia seeds (optional)

1 teaspoon vanilla extract

PROCESS:

Stir all ingredients together in a medium bowl until thoroughly mixed. Cover and let chill in the refrigerator for half an hour. Once chilled, roll into balls of whatever size you would like. (Mine are about 1″ in diameter.) Store in an airtight container and keep refrigerated for up to 1 week. Makes about 20-25 balls.

BEET KVASS

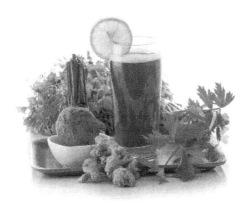

I have no doubt that you're scratching your head right now and saying, "What in the world is beet kvass?" This is one of my most recent discoveries and while I can't yet testify of its long-term effects, I can tell you that it has proven itself to be a powerful detoxifier. So, for those of you who are ready to REALLY clean out your body and improve your overall health, this one is for you. It's definitely an acquired taste, but the

health benefits are so noticeable that even
my dog looks forward to his daily dose.

INGREDIENTS:
Filtered water
3-4 beets
1 ½ tablespoon unrefined sea salt
¼ cup juice from sauerkraut or pickles
(optional)

PROCESS:
Wash the beets of any dirt, but do not scrub
or peel the beets.
Chop the beets. Do not shred.
Add the beets to a 1-gallon jar.
Add sea salt and juice (if using).
Add filtered water to ½ inch below lid
Affix lid tightly and label with date.
Allow to ferment for 2 days (if using juice) or
1 week (if only using salt)out of direct
sunlight. You'll know the juice is ready when
the liquid is bubbling on the top like a
carbonated drink.
Strain and then store in the refrigerator, or
feel free to store in the refrigerator as is.

NOTE:

I have found that I like using starter cultures better than juice or plain salt. I found mine on Amazon for a very reasonable price. As for the process itself, I do mine a little differently in that I divide my ingredients up over four quart-sized jars and allow them to ferment like that. Once the fermentation is complete, I strain them into a gallon-size glass jar with a spout. This makes it easy to get my daily supply without a lot of hassle. If the taste is really more than you can handle, try mixing it with a fruit juice that is 100% juice. Start with half and half, then work your way down.

Also, you can ferment other fruits, vegetables and spices with your beets to come up with your own original concoctions. My favorite so far is my citrus/ginger beet kvass, which uses shredded ginger root, orange, lemon, lime and, of course, beets.

RISE UP AND BUILD

SUPER DETOX GREENS SMOOTHIE

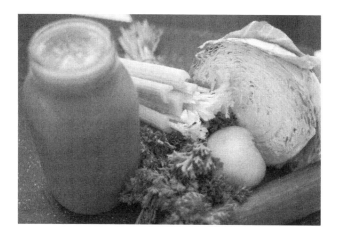

Okay, this is another recipe for those who
are fearless and dedicated. This smoothie
is very filling and works well as a breakfast
replacement. I won't say that it's the best
thing I've ever tasted, but it does have a
very refreshing taste.

INGREDIENTS:

1 cup spinach or kale leaves

1 cup romaine leaves

½ cup chopped cucumber

½ cup chopped celery

1 small pear (or ½ large), cored and chopped

1 banana, chopped (preferably frozen)

1 cup water or coconut water

1 tablespoon of fresh mint

1 tablespoon of fresh parsley

½ to 1 whole lemon, juiced

½ tablespoon chia seeds

¼-inch slice ginger root, peeled

pinch of cayenne, optional

pinch of cinnamon, optional

pinch of turmeric, optional

PROCESS:

Place the ingredients in a blender and blend until completely smooth. If it's not sweet enough, you can add a touch of honey, molasses or maple syrup.

RISE UP AND BUILD RESOURCES

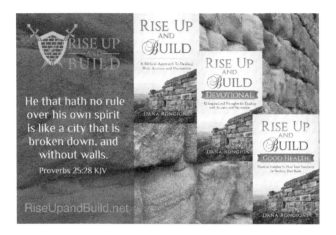

If you enjoyed this book and would like to find out more about dealing with anxiety and depression, I encourage you to pick up the other books in the series: **Rise Up and Build** and **Rise Up and Build Devotional**. Each of these books build on the principles established in this book, giving you resources to heal your body, mind and spirit.

If you're looking for additional ways to combat anxiety and depression, I invite you to visit RiseUpandBuild.net, where you'll find numerous free resources to aid you in your battle toward freedom.

ABOUT THE AUTHOR

Dana Rongione is the author of several Christian books, including the highly-praised *Giggles and Grace* devotional series for women. A dedicated wife and doggie "mom," Dana lives in Greenville, SC, where she spends her days writing and reaching out to the hurting and discouraged. Connect with her on her website, DanaRongione.com, and be sure to sign up for her daily devotions.

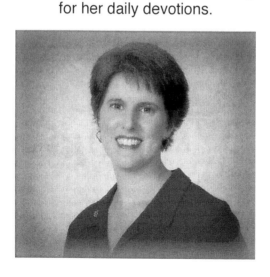

BOOKS BY DANA RONGIONE

Devotional/Christian Living:

He's Still Working Miracles: Daring To Ask God for the Impossible

There's a Verse for That

'Paws'itively Divine: Devotions for Dog Lovers

The Deadly Darts of the Devil

What Happened To Prince Charming?: Ten Tips to Achieve a Happy Marriage Life and Live Happily Ever After

Rise Up and Build Devotional: 52 Inspirational Thoughts for Dealing with Anxiety and Depression

Giggles and Grace Series:

Random Ramblings of a Raving Redhead

Daily Discussions of a Doubting Disciple

Lilting Laments of a Looney Lass

Mindful Musings of a Moody Motivator

Other Titles for Adults:

Rise Up and Build: A Biblical Approach To Dealing With Anxiety and Depression

Rise Up and Build Good Health: Practical Insights to Heal Your Emotions by Healing Your Body

Creating a World of Your Own: Your Guide to Writing Fiction

The Delaware Detectives Middle-Grade Mystery Series:

Book #1 – The Delaware Detectives: A Middle-Grade Mystery

Book #2 – Through Many Dangers

Book #3 – My Fears Relieved

Book #4 – I Once Was Lost

Books for Young Children:

Through the Eyes of a Child

God Can Use My Differences

Audio Bible Studies:

Moodswing Mania – a Bible study through select Psalms (6 CD's)

The Names of God – a 6-CD Bible study exploring some of the most powerful names of God

Miracles of the Old Testament, Part 1 – a Bible study with a unique look at miracles in the Old Testament (4 CD's)

There's a Verse for That – Scripture with a soft music background, perfect for meditation or memorization

ACKNOWLEDGMENTS

This book would not have been possible without the help and support of the following people:

The Lord, my Strength and Song — Without Him, I can do nothing!

My husband, Jason

My loyal and high-ranking patrons:
>Lewis and Sharon White
>Patty Hicks
>Dawn Hodge
>Jo Anne Hall
>Peter Santaniello
>Lisa Gutschow
>Tara Looper
>And others who wish to remain anonymous. . .

My church family who constantly asked, "When will the new book be ready?" They urged me to complete the task, no matter how overwhelming it seemed at times.

RISE UP AND BUILD

`

Made in the USA
Middletown, DE
19 July 2021